TOWARD
Healthy Living

A Wellness Journal

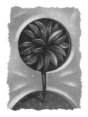

An Official Publication
of the Arthritis Foundation
ATLANTA, GEORGIA

Published by
Arthritis Foundation
1330 West Peachtree St.
Atlanta, GA 30309

Printed in the United States of America
1st printing 1997

ISBN: 1-56352-453-8

EDITORIAL DIRECTOR: Adrienne Greer
PRODUCTION DIRECTOR: Elizabeth Compton
ART DIRECTOR: Jennifer Rogers
COVER ILLUSTRATION: Mark Bender

Special thanks to the following individuals for their help with this project:
Janet Austin, PhD, Doyt L. Conn, MD, Cathay Loadman, Cindy McDaniel, Shelly Morrow,
Bill Otto, Susan Percy, Jarred Schenke and Michele Taylor of the Arthritis Foundation;
plus Chuck Perry and others at Longstreet Press.

"Afoot and light-hearted I take to the open road,

Healthy, free, the world before me,

The long brown path before me leading wherever I choose."

From "Song of the Open Road,"
by Walt Whitman

OUR MISSION

The mission of the Arthritis Foundation is to support research to find the cure for and prevention of arthritis and to improve the quality of life for those affected by arthritis.

FOREWORD

Journaling is an age-old method of documenting important events or moments. As a child, you may have written special thoughts inside a diary then clasped its metal lock shut so no one would see; aviators have long recorded travel patterns and weather conditions in travel logs; cooks scribble ingredients and instructions in recipe books. Even the medical records your doctor keeps in his office serve as a journal of sorts, recording visits and important information about your health-care treatment and management.

If you are affected by a type of arthritis or one of the 100-plus arthritis-related conditions, you may find that keeping a journal is an easy, rewarding and proactive way to take part in your health care. In each of its self-help courses – for arthritis, fibromyalgia and lupus – the Arthritis Foundation endorses journaling as an important activity that provides a creative outlet for venting feelings or thoughts that may accompany your condition. By journaling, you are able to process your symptoms, feelings and thoughts and free your mind to focus on healing.

Toward Healthy Living – A Wellness Journal explains the benefits of keeping a journal, and suggests ways to organize your thoughts. Use the pages as a thoughts diary to record pleasant or unpleasant emotions you're experiencing and to note how you feel physically as a result. Monitor your pain and mood levels to learn more about possible associations between the two. Keep track of your exercise activities – how much and how often – and what impact they have on the way you feel.

The key to living well with arthritis – or any arthritis-related disease or condition – is taking an active role in your own health-care treatment. *Toward Healthy Living – A Wellness Journal* is a tool created by the Arthritis Foundation to help you do just that.

DOYT L. CONN, M.D.
Senior Vice President, Medical Affairs
Arthritis Foundation

INTRODUCTION

You have purchased this journal because you want to take charge of your life. When you live with the long-term pain, limitations and fatigue that accompany osteoarthritis, fibromyalgia, lupus, rheumatoid arthritis, gout or any other chronic condition, it's sometimes easy to become passive, allowing others to make decisions and do things for you. But that could be a critical mistake. Living well with chronic pain and illness begins with action, first by learning about your condition, then by doing something about it.

Keeping a journal is a practical, yet personal, approach. A journal by most standards is a book in which to write your innermost private thoughts. It is also a ledger of sorts, a place in which to record things you want to keep or need to remember.

The Arthritis Foundation combined these two ideas to create *Toward Healthy Living – A Wellness Journal.* This book is designed with you in mind, providing ample pages where you can unleash your thoughts, and designated spaces ideal for monitoring your pain and moods. Jot down your thoughts on the pages, then close the book and leave them inside.

Throughout this book, you'll find wisdom from a variety of people – those who live with chronic pain and illness, and those who don't. Read their words for what they're worth, then add your own words of inspiration to the adjacent pages.

Finally, the Arthritis Foundation has included a comprehensive listing of resources to which you may refer from time to time. In the spaces provided, add names and numbers of new resources you come across.

Why Keep a Journal?

In *Opening Up: The Healing Power of Confiding in Others,* James Pennebaker explains that people with chronic illness who write about their painful feelings and losses in some type of journal report fewer symptoms, fewer visits to the doctor, fewer days off work, improved mood and outlook, and even enhanced immune function.

Keeping records of your experiences with your condition can make a difference in your health. Many people find it useful to write them in a journal, and some find it helpful to share them with their physician or other health-care providers. A written record of your experiences can:

- provide you with concrete documentation of your symptoms
- help you communicate with your doctors and other health-care providers
- help you explain your situation to family, friends, co-workers or employers
- help you understand your disease more fully and identify your symptom patterns throughout the year
- help you identify factors that trigger symptoms and fluctuations
- provide you with an objective memory aid
- help you "process" your symptoms, feelings and thoughts, and let them go, freeing your mind to focus on healing
- help you re-assert control.

As you begin recording your symptoms and experiences, monitor only what is important to you – not what you think you ought to care about. Consider the following factors as you write in your journal:

- unusual symptoms
- stress or frustrations
- exercise participation
- activity level
- positive changes
- mood changes
- thoughts and reactions to daily events
- something funny you saw or heard.

Keeping a journal, like any new habit, may take a while to feel natural. To give it a fair trial, set a schedule, such as writing for five to 10 minutes, three times a week. If you like it, you'll probably find yourself writing on a regular basis.

Select a method that fits your schedule and needs. Here are a few strategies:

- Keep a running log of your symptoms. Enter symptoms daily or weekly as needed during flares or times of uncertainty.

- Write about your experiences with your condition and your reactions to these experiences. Don't just record what happened, but describe how you felt when it happened.

- Consider dividing your journal page in half. Record all of the "facts" of the day – problems, challenges or positive experiences – on one side. On the other side, record your emotional reactions to and thoughts about these events. Logs like these are useful for emotional release as well as for self-discovery.

- Select only a few symptoms to monitor initially, such as your pain level, fatigue and mood. You may want to keep track of how your symptoms change. By doing so, you can see the interrelationships among these symptoms over time.

- Date your entries so that you can look back over them and see patterns and progress.

- Write freely and selfishly. Don't worry about grammar or misspellings. You may want to keep this diary to yourself – some people find they write more honestly that way. Write to develop insight into your feelings – it can be an emotional release. But don't write to avoid taking needed action.

Take Charge of Your Life

People who successfully manage their lives with chronic illness have found innumerable, ingenious methods of dealing with their conditions. Keeping a journal is just one popular example. The key to living well with any chronic condition is leading a healthy life – despite your disease. That includes finding a balance between exercise and rest, eating a nutritious diet, and nourishing your mind and spirit, as well as your body. It is our hope that this journal will serve as a compass on your journey toward healthy living.

Arthritis Foundation

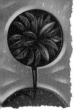

DATE _____

_____
_____
_____
_____
_____
_____

"You are every-
thing that is –
your thoughts,
your life, your
dreams come
true. You are
everything you
choose to be.
You are as un-
limited as the
endless universe."

Shad Helmstetter,
psychologist
and author

_____
_____
_____
_____
_____
_____
_____
_____
_____
_____
_____
_____
_____
_____
_____
_____
_____
_____

My mood today was:						My level of pain today was:					
0	1	2	3	4	5	0	1	2	3	4	5
GOOD					BAD	MILD					SEVERE

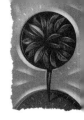

DATE

My mood today was:

0	1	2	3	4	5

GOOD ———————————————— BAD

My level of pain today was:

0	1	2	3	4	5

MILD ———————————————— SEVERE

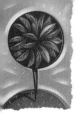

DATE _____

_____

_____

_____

_____

_____

_____

_____

_____

_____

_____

_____

_____

_____

_____

_____

_____

_____

_____

_____

_____

_____

_____

_____

_____

| My mood today was: |
| 0   1   2   3   4   5 |
| GOOD ———————————— BAD |

| My level of pain today was: |
| 0   1   2   3   4   5 |
| MILD ———————————— SEVERE |

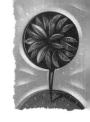

DATE

_____

—————————————————————————————————
—————————————————————————————————
—————————————————————————————————
—————————————————————————————————
—————————————————————————————————
—————————————————————————————————
—————————————————————————————————

*"As we expand
our lives and do
things that are
challenging, in-
novative and
unpredictable,
we can know
what it means
to be filled with
joy and the peace
that passes un-
derstanding."*

From **Living Faith,**
by Jimmy Carter,
39th President of
the United States

My mood today was:					
0	1	2	3	4	5
GOOD					BAD

My level of pain today was:					
0	1	2	3	4	5
MILD					SEVERE

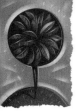

DATE _____

_____

_____

_____

_____

_____

_____

_____

"Self-pity in its
early stages is as
snug as a feather
mattress. Only
when it hardens
does it become
uncomfortable."

From *Gather*
Together in
My Name, by
Maya Angelou,
poet and author

_____

_____

_____

_____

_____

_____

_____

_____

_____

_____

_____

_____

_____

_____

_____

My mood today was:							My level of pain today was:					
0	1	2	3	4	5		0	1	2	3	4	5
GOOD					BAD		MILD					SEVERE

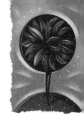

_____ DATE

_____

_____
_____
_____
_____
_____
_____
_____
_____
_____
_____
_____
_____
_____
_____
_____
_____
_____
_____
_____
_____
_____
_____
_____
_____
_____
_____
_____
_____
_____

My mood today was:							**My level of pain today was:**					
0	1	2	3	4	5		0	1	2	3	4	5
GOOD					BAD		MILD					SEVERE

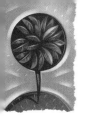

DATE

_____

_____

_____

_____

_____

_____

_____

_____

_____

_____

_____

_____

_____

_____

_____

_____

_____

_____

_____

_____

_____

_____

_____

_____

_____

_____

_____

My mood today was:					
0	1	2	3	4	5
GOOD					BAD

My level of pain today was:					
0	1	2	3	4	5
MILD					SEVERE

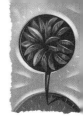

_____

_____
_____
_____
_____
_____
_____
_____
_____
_____
_____
_____
_____
_____
_____
_____
_____
_____
_____
_____
_____
_____
_____

"Exercise #15
1. Have fun today.
2. Do it again
tomorrow."

From **To Lead**
is to Serve,
by Shar McBee

My mood today was:

0	1	2	3	4	5
GOOD					BAD

My level of pain today was:

0	1	2	3	4	5
MILD					SEVERE

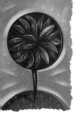

DATE _____

_____

_____

_____

_____

_____

_____

_____

_____

_____

"Where I was born _____
and where and
how I have lived _____
is unimportant.
It is what I _____
have done with
where I have _____
been that should
be of interest." _____

Georgia O'Keeffe, _____
American artist
_____

_____

_____

_____

_____

_____

_____

_____

_____

My mood today was:					
0	1	2	3	4	5
GOOD					BAD

My level of pain today was:					
0	1	2	3	4	5
MILD					SEVERE

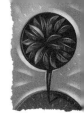

DATE _____

_____

_____

_____

_____

_____

_____

_____

_____

_____

_____

_____

_____

_____

_____

_____

_____

_____

_____

_____

_____

_____

_____

_____

_____

_____

My mood today was:

0	1	2	3	4	5

GOOD ———————————————— BAD

My level of pain today was:

0	1	2	3	4	5

MILD ———————————————— SEVERE

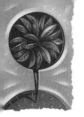

DATE _____

_____

_____

_____

_____

_____

_____

_____

_____

_____

_____

_____

_____

_____

_____

_____

_____

_____

_____

_____

_____

_____

_____

_____

_____

_____

_____

_____

_____

My mood today was:

0	1	2	3	4	5

GOOD ———————————————— BAD

My level of pain today was:

0	1	2	3	4	5

MILD ———————————————— SEVERE

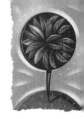

_____

_____

_____

_____

_____

_____

_____

_____

"Everything that is done in the world is done by hope."

Martin Luther, German theologian and leader of the Protestant Reformation in Germany

_____

_____

_____

_____

_____

_____

_____

_____

_____

_____

_____

_____

_____

_____

My mood today was:

0	1	2	3	4	5
GOOD					BAD

My level of pain today was:

0	1	2	3	4	5
MILD					SEVERE

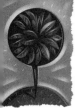

DATE _____

_____
_____
_____
_____
_____
_____
_____

"The best remedy
for those who are
afraid, lonely or
unhappy is to
go outside, some-
where where they
can be quite
alone with the
heavens, nature
and God. I firmly
believe that nature
brings solace in
all troubles."

From *Diary of*
a Young Girl,
by Anne Frank

_____
_____
_____
_____
_____
_____
_____
_____
_____
_____
_____
_____
_____
_____
_____

My mood today was:					
0	1	2	3	4	5
GOOD					BAD

My level of pain today was:					
0	1	2	3	4	5
MILD					SEVERE

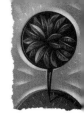

DATE

_____

_____

_____

_____

_____

_____

_____

_____

_____

_____

_____

_____

_____

_____

_____

_____

_____

_____

_____

_____

_____

_____

_____

_____

_____

My mood today was:

| 0 | 1 | 2 | 3 | 4 | 5 |

GOOD ———————————————— BAD

My level of pain today was:

| 0 | 1 | 2 | 3 | 4 | 5 |

MILD ———————————————— SEVERE

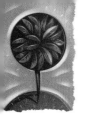

DATE

My mood today was:

| 0 | 1 | 2 | 3 | 4 | 5 |

GOOD ——————————————— BAD

My level of pain today was:

| 0 | 1 | 2 | 3 | 4 | 5 |

MILD ——————————————— SEVERE

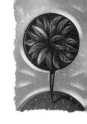

DATE

_____

"*The wild things roared their terrible roars and gnashed their terrible teeth and rolled their terrible eyes and showed their terrible claws but Max stepped into his private boat and waved goodbye.*"

From *Where the Wild Things Are,* by Maurice Sendak

My mood today was:

0	1	2	3	4	5
GOOD					BAD

My level of pain today was:

0	1	2	3	4	5
MILD					SEVERE

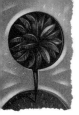

DATE _____

_____
_____
_____
_____
_____
_____
_____

*"The vision that
you glorify in
your mind, the
ideal that you
enthrone in your
heart – this you
will build your
life by, this you
will become."*

From Dorothy
Hulst's *As a Woman
Thinketh,* a tran-
scription for women
of James Allen's
famous essay *As a
Man Thinketh.*

_____
_____
_____
_____
_____
_____
_____
_____
_____
_____
_____
_____
_____
_____
_____
_____
_____

My mood today was:						My level of pain today was:					
0	1	2	3	4	5	0	1	2	3	4	5
GOOD					BAD	MILD					SEVERE

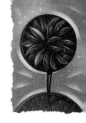

DATE _____

_____

_____
_____
_____
_____
_____
_____
_____
_____
_____
_____
_____
_____
_____
_____
_____
_____
_____
_____
_____
_____
_____
_____
_____
_____
_____
_____
_____
_____
_____

My mood today was:

0	1	2	3	4	5
GOOD					BAD

My level of pain today was:

0	1	2	3	4	5
MILD					SEVERE

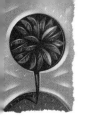

DATE _____

_____

_____

_____

_____

_____

_____

_____

_____

_____

_____

_____

_____

_____

_____

_____

_____

_____

_____

_____

_____

_____

_____

_____

_____

_____

My mood today was:							**My level of pain today was:**					
0	1	2	3	4	5		0	1	2	3	4	5
GOOD					BAD		MILD					SEVERE

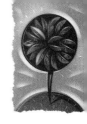

DATE _____

_____

_____

_____

_____

_____

_____

_____

_____   *"Learn from*
                                                          yesterday.
_____   *Live for today.*

_____   *Look to tomorrow.*

_____   *Rest this*
                                                          afternoon."
_____

_____   Wisdom from
                                                          Snoopy in **Life's**
_____   **Answers,** by
                                                          Charles M. Schulz
_____

_____

_____

_____

_____

_____

_____

_____

_____

_____

My mood today was:							My level of pain today was:					
0	1	2	3	4	5		0	1	2	3	4	5
GOOD					BAD		MILD					SEVERE

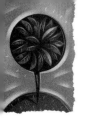

DATE _____

_____
_____
_____
_____
_____
_____
_____

*"Isn't it a bit
unnerving
that doctors
call what they
do 'practice'?"*

Unknown

_____
_____
_____
_____
_____
_____
_____
_____
_____
_____
_____
_____
_____
_____

My mood today was:					
0	1	2	3	4	5
GOOD					BAD

My level of pain today was:					
0	1	2	3	4	5
MILD					SEVERE

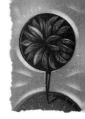

DATE

_____

_____
_____
_____
_____
_____
_____
_____
_____
_____
_____
_____
_____
_____
_____
_____
_____
_____
_____
_____
_____
_____
_____
_____
_____
_____
_____
_____

My mood today was:

0	1	2	3	4	5
GOOD					BAD

My level of pain today was:

0	1	2	3	4	5
MILD					SEVERE

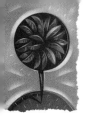

DATE _____

_____

_____

_____

_____

_____

_____

_____

_____

_____

_____

_____

_____

_____

_____

_____

_____

_____

_____

_____

_____

_____

_____

_____

_____

_____

_____

My mood today was:					
0	1	2	3	4	5
GOOD					BAD

My level of pain today was:					
0	1	2	3	4	5
MILD					SEVERE

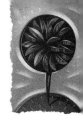

_____

_____

_____

_____

_____

_____

_____

_____

_____

_____   *"You gain strength,*
                                        courage and
_____   *confidence by*
                                        every experience
_____   *in which you*
                                        really stop to look
_____   *fear in the face."*

_____   Eleanor Roosevelt,
                                        writer, United
_____   Nations delegate
                                        and wife of Franklin
_____   D. Roosevelt, 32nd
                                        President of the
_____   United States

_____

_____

_____

_____

_____

_____

_____

My mood today was:						My level of pain today was:					
0	1	2	3	4	5	0	1	2	3	4	5
GOOD					BAD	MILD					SEVERE

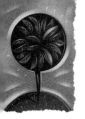

DATE _____

_____
_____
_____
_____
_____
_____
_____
_____
_____
_____
_____
_____
_____
_____
_____
_____
_____
_____
_____
_____
_____
_____
_____
_____
_____
_____
_____

"I have come to feel that dying is the easy part, the breathing out of the spirit, for it requires no effort. The real challenge lies in grieving my losses and then turning back to a life complicated by chronic illness, rejoicing in the daily celebration of the gift of that life – the joy-dance of present moment living!"

From *Successful Living with Chronic Illness – Celebrating the Joys of Life,* by Kathleen Lewis, single mother of two who lives with lupus and fibromyalgia

My mood today was:						My level of pain today was:					
0	1	2	3	4	5	0	1	2	3	4	5
GOOD					BAD	MILD					SEVERE

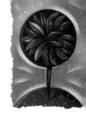

_____ DATE

_____

_____
_____
_____
_____
_____
_____
_____
_____
_____
_____
_____
_____
_____
_____
_____
_____
_____
_____
_____
_____
_____
_____
_____
_____
_____
_____

My mood today was:

0	1	2	3	4	5
GOOD					BAD

My level of pain today was:

0	1	2	3	4	5
MILD					SEVERE

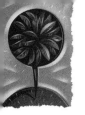

DATE _____

_____

_____

_____

_____

_____

_____

_____

_____

_____

_____

_____

_____

_____

_____

_____

_____

_____

_____

_____

_____

_____

_____

_____

_____

_____

My mood today was:	**My level of pain today was:**
0 1 2 3 4 5	0 1 2 3 4 5
GOOD ———————————— BAD	MILD ———————————— SEVERE

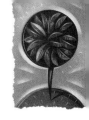

"...as long as there is joy in creation there will always be new creations to discover, or to rediscover, and a prime place to look is within and about the self."

Alice Walker, Pulitzer Prize-winning author, from a talk she gave at Spelman College in Atlanta, Ga.

My mood today was:

0	1	2	3	4	5
GOOD					BAD

My level of pain today was:

0	1	2	3	4	5
MILD					SEVERE

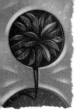

DATE _____

_____
_____
_____
_____
_____
_____
_____

"Life only demands
from you the
strength you pos-
sess. Only one feat
is possible – not to
have run away."

Dag Hammarskjold,
Swedish statesman,
Nobel Peace Prize
winner and former
secretary general of
the United Nations

_____
_____
_____
_____
_____
_____
_____
_____
_____
_____
_____
_____
_____
_____
_____
_____
_____

My mood today was:

0	1	2	3	4	5
GOOD					BAD

My level of pain today was:

0	1	2	3	4	5
MILD					SEVERE

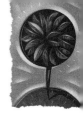

DATE _____

_____

_____

_____

_____

_____

_____

_____

_____

_____

_____

_____

_____

_____

_____

_____

_____

_____

_____

_____

_____

_____

_____

_____

My mood today was:	**My level of pain today was:**
0　1　2　3　4　5	0　1　2　3　4　5
GOOD ——————————— BAD	MILD ——————————— SEVERE

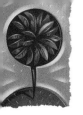

DATE _____

_____
_____
_____
_____
_____
_____
_____
_____
_____
_____
_____
_____
_____
_____
_____
_____
_____
_____
_____
_____
_____
_____
_____
_____
_____
_____

My mood today was:

0	1	2	3	4	5
GOOD					BAD

My level of pain today was:

0	1	2	3	4	5
MILD					SEVERE

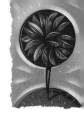

"If I can help some-body as I pass along, if I can cheer somebody with a word and a song, if I can show somebody he's traveling wrong, then my living will not in be vain."

Nobel Peace Prize winner and civil rights leader Dr. Martin Luther King, Jr., from a sermon he preached several weeks before he died; it was played at his funeral

My mood today was:

0	1	2	3	4	5
GOOD					BAD

My level of pain today was:

0	1	2	3	4	5
MILD					SEVERE

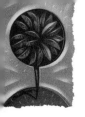

DATE _____

_____

_____

_____

_____

_____

_____

_____

"Sure, I'm for
helping the elderly.
I'm going to be old
myself someday."   _____

_____

Lillian Carter,
mother of Jimmy   _____
Carter, 39th
President of the   _____
United States
_____

_____

_____

_____

_____

_____

_____

_____

_____

_____

_____

_____

_____

My mood today was:	**My level of pain today was:**
0 1 2 3 4 5	0 1 2 3 4 5
GOOD ——————— BAD	MILD ——————— SEVERE

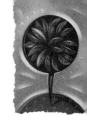

DATE _____

_____

_____

_____

_____

_____

_____

_____

_____

_____

_____

_____

_____

_____

_____

_____

_____

_____

_____

_____

_____

_____

_____

_____

_____

_____

_____

My mood today was:		**My level of pain today was:**
0 1 2 3 4 5		0 1 2 3 4 5
GOOD ———————————— BAD		MILD ———————————— SEVERE

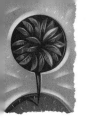

DATE _____

_____

_____

_____

_____

_____

_____

_____

_____

_____

_____

_____

_____

_____

_____

_____

_____

_____

_____

_____

_____

_____

_____

_____

_____

My mood today was:							**My level of pain today was:**					
0	1	2	3	4	5		0	1	2	3	4	5
GOOD					BAD		MILD					SEVERE

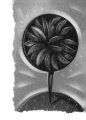

DATE

"*Obstacles are
those frightening
things you see
when you take
your eyes off
your goal.*"

Henry Ford,
American automo-
bile manufacturer

My mood today was:					
0	1	2	3	4	5
GOOD					BAD

My level of pain today was:					
0	1	2	3	4	5
MILD					SEVERE

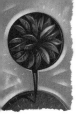

DATE

"*Once you learn to
live with arthritis
in a way that you
see some good out
of it, then you've
begun to heal.*"

Former gymnast and
1960 Olympian Tuovi
Cochrane of Rock-
ford, Mich. Cochrane
has rheumatoid
arthritis. As quoted in
Arthritis Today
July-August 1996

My mood today was:					
0	1	2	3	4	5
GOOD					BAD

My level of pain today was:					
0	1	2	3	4	5
MILD					SEVERE

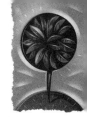

DATE _____

_____

_____

_____

_____

_____

_____

_____

_____

_____

_____

_____

_____

_____

_____

_____

_____

_____

_____

_____

_____

_____

_____

_____

_____

_____

_____

_____

_____

My mood today was:

0	1	2	3	4	5
GOOD					BAD

My level of pain today was:

0	1	2	3	4	5
MILD					SEVERE

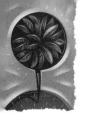

DATE _____

_____
_____
_____
_____
_____
_____
_____
_____
_____
_____
_____
_____
_____
_____
_____
_____
_____
_____
_____
_____
_____
_____
_____
_____

My mood today was:						My level of pain today was:					
0	1	2	3	4	5	0	1	2	3	4	5
GOOD					BAD	MILD					SEVERE

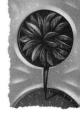

"*All the good stories are out there waiting to be told in a fresh, wild way.*"

From *Bird by Bird,* by Anne Lamott

My mood today was:					
0	1	2	3	4	5
GOOD					BAD

My level of pain today was:					
0	1	2	3	4	5
MILD					SEVERE

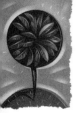

DATE _____

_____

_____

_____

_____

_____

_____

_____

"I am bigger than
anything that
can happen to me.
All these things,
sorrow, misfortune,
and suffering, are
outside my door.
I am in the house
and I have a key."

Charles Fletcher
Lummis, South-
western author,
librarian, historian
and archaeologist

_____

_____

_____

_____

_____

_____

_____

_____

_____

_____

_____

_____

_____

My mood today was:						**My level of pain today was:**					
0	1	2	3	4	5	0	1	2	3	4	5
GOOD					BAD	MILD					SEVERE

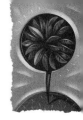

DATE

My mood today was:

0   1   2   3   4   5

GOOD ————————————— BAD

My level of pain today was:

0   1   2   3   4   5

MILD ————————————— SEVERE

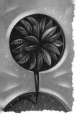

DATE

_____

_____

_____

_____

_____

_____

_____

_____

_____

_____

_____

_____

_____

_____

_____

_____

_____

_____

_____

_____

_____

_____

_____

My mood today was:							My level of pain today was:					
0	1	2	3	4	5		0	1	2	3	4	5
GOOD					BAD		MILD					SEVERE

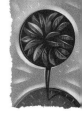

---

*"He who laughs
last, thinks
slowest."*

Unknown

My mood today was:

0	1	2	3	4	5
GOOD					BAD

My level of pain today was:

0	1	2	3	4	5
MILD					SEVERE

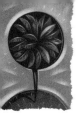

DATE

"There is only one corner of the universe you can be certain of improving, and that's your own self."

Aldous Huxley, English novelist and essayist

My mood today was:

0	1	2	3	4	5
GOOD					BAD

My level of pain today was:

0	1	2	3	4	5
MILD					SEVERE

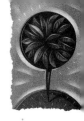

DATE

_____

_____

_____

_____

_____

_____

_____

_____

_____

_____

_____

_____

_____

_____

_____

_____

_____

_____

_____

_____

_____

_____

_____

_____

_____

_____

My mood today was:						My level of pain today was:					
0	1	2	3	4	5	0	1	2	3	4	5
GOOD					BAD	MILD					SEVERE

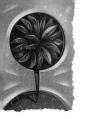

DATE _____

_____

_____

_____

_____

_____

_____

_____

_____

_____

_____

_____

_____

_____

_____

_____

_____

_____

_____

_____

_____

_____

_____

_____

_____

My mood today was:						My level of pain today was:					
0	1	2	3	4	5	0	1	2	3	4	5
GOOD					BAD	MILD					SEVERE

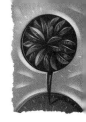

DATE

"Our imagination is the only limit to what we can hope to have in the future."

Charles F. Kettering, American electrical engineer and inventor

My mood today was:

0 1 2 3 4 5

GOOD ————————————————— BAD

My level of pain today was:

0 1 2 3 4 5

MILD ————————————————— SEVERE

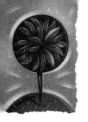

DATE _____

_____

_____

_____

_____

_____

_____

_____

_____

*"We come to feel
as we behave."*

Paul Pearsall,
author

_____

_____

_____

_____

_____

_____

_____

_____

_____

_____

_____

_____

_____

My mood today was:						**My level of pain today was:**					
0	1	2	3	4	5	0	1	2	3	4	5
GOOD					BAD	MILD					SEVERE

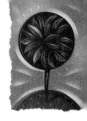

DATE _____

_____

_____

_____

_____

_____

_____

_____

_____

_____

_____

_____

_____

_____

_____

_____

_____

_____

_____

_____

_____

_____

_____

_____

_____

_____

_____

_____

My mood today was:

0	1	2	3	4	5

GOOD ————————————————— BAD

My level of pain today was:

0	1	2	3	4	5

MILD ————————————————— SEVERE

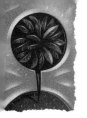

DATE _____

_____
_____
_____
_____
_____
_____
_____
_____
_____
_____
_____
_____
_____
_____
_____
_____
_____
_____
_____
_____
_____
_____
_____
_____

	My mood today was:						**My level of pain today was:**				
0	1	2	3	4	5	0	1	2	3	4	5
GOOD					BAD	MILD					SEVERE

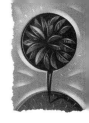

_____

_____

_____

_____

_____

_____

_____

_____

_____

_____

_____

_____

_____

_____

_____

_____

_____

_____

_____

_____

_____

_____

_____

_____

_____

_____

_____

_____

_____

_____

_____

_____

"The pain [of arthritis] has really opened my eyes to see the pain in the world in general. It's made me more sensitive to other people. I'm a much better, a much stronger person than I would have been otherwise, and I want to use those qualities to make life a little better for others."

Tom Juneman, reflecting on his acceptance of a diagnosis of rheumatoid arthritis, which followed bouts of denial. As quoted in *Arthritis Today,* July-August 1992

My mood today was:

0	1	2	3	4	5

GOOD ——————————————— BAD

My level of pain today was:

0	1	2	3	4	5

MILD ——————————————— SEVERE

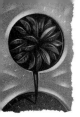

DATE _____

_____

_____

_____

_____

_____

_____

"Of any stopping
place in life,
it is good to ask
whether it will be
a good place
from which to go
as well as a good
place to remain."

From **Composing a**
Life, by professor
and writer Mary
Catherine Bateson

_____

_____

_____

_____

_____

_____

_____

_____

_____

_____

_____

_____

_____

_____

My mood today was:						My level of pain today was:					
0	1	2	3	4	5	0	1	2	3	4	5
GOOD					BAD	MILD					SEVERE

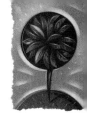

DATE

My mood today was:

0	1	2	3	4	5

GOOD ———————————————— BAD

My level of pain today was:

0	1	2	3	4	5

MILD ———————————————— SEVERE

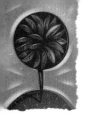

DATE _____

_____

_____

_____

_____

_____

_____

_____

_____

_____

_____

_____

_____

_____

_____

_____

_____

_____

_____

_____

_____

_____

_____

_____

_____

_____

My mood today was:

0	1	2	3	4	5

GOOD ———————————————— BAD

My level of pain today was:

0	1	2	3	4	5

MILD ———————————————— SEVERE

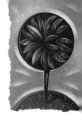

DATE _____

_____

_____
_____
_____
_____
_____
_____
_____
_____

"Generations of
Americans have
escaped pain by
crawling inside
a banana split
and pulling the
ice cream shut
behind them."

From a menu at
Sweeney Todd's
Cafe in London

_____
_____
_____
_____
_____
_____
_____
_____
_____
_____
_____

My mood today was:

0	1	2	3	4	5
GOOD					BAD

My level of pain today was:

0	1	2	3	4	5
MILD					SEVERE

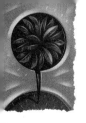

DATE _____

_____

_____

_____

_____

_____

_____

"I don't suffer from insanity, I enjoy every minute of it."

Bumper sticker

_____

_____

_____

_____

_____

_____

_____

_____

_____

_____

_____

_____

_____

_____

_____

_____

My mood today was:					
0	1	2	3	4	5
GOOD					BAD

My level of pain today was:					
0	1	2	3	4	5
MILD					SEVERE

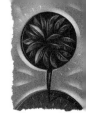

DATE _____

_____

_____

_____

_____

_____

_____

_____

_____

_____

_____

_____

_____

_____

_____

_____

_____

_____

_____

_____

_____

_____

_____

_____

_____

My mood today was:	**My level of pain today was:**
0 1 2 3 4 5	0 1 2 3 4 5
GOOD ——————————— BAD	MILD ——————————— SEVERE

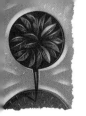

DATE _____

_____
_____
_____
_____
_____
_____
_____
_____
_____
_____
_____
_____
_____
_____
_____
_____
_____
_____
_____
_____
_____
_____
_____
_____
_____
_____

My mood today was:

0	1	2	3	4	5

GOOD ———————————————— BAD

My level of pain today was:

0	1	2	3	4	5

MILD ———————————————— SEVERE

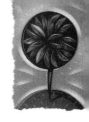

_____

_____

_____

_____

_____

_____

_____

_____

_____

_____

_____

_____

_____

_____

_____

_____

_____

_____

_____

_____

_____

_____

_____

_____

"A handicap is only a handicap when it ceases to be a challenge."

Submitted by **Arthritis Today** reader Carlyn Creel of Weaver, Ala., who heard a minister use this quote in a sermon on the radio. Creel has rheumatoid arthritis.

My mood today was:

0	1	2	3	4	5
GOOD					BAD

My level of pain today was:

0	1	2	3	4	5
MILD					SEVERE

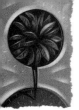

DATE _____

_____

_____

_____

_____

_____

_____

*"You have brains
in your head.*

*You have feet in
your shoes.*

*You can steer
yourself any
direction you
choose."*

From *Oh the
Places You'll Go,*
by Dr. Seuss
(Theodor Geisel)

_____

_____

_____

_____

_____

_____

_____

_____

_____

_____

_____

_____

_____

_____

My mood today was:					
0	1	2	3	4	5
GOOD					BAD

My level of pain today was:					
0	1	2	3	4	5
MILD					SEVERE

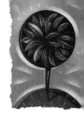

DATE

_____

My mood today was:

| 0 | 1 | 2 | 3 | 4 | 5 |

GOOD ——————————————— BAD

My level of pain today was:

| 0 | 1 | 2 | 3 | 4 | 5 |

MILD ——————————————— SEVERE

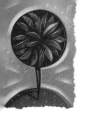

DATE _____

_____

_____

_____

_____

_____

_____

_____

_____

_____

_____

_____

_____

_____

_____

_____

_____

_____

_____

_____

_____

_____

_____

_____

_____

_____

My mood today was:							**My level of pain today was:**					
0	1	2	3	4	5		0	1	2	3	4	5
GOOD					BAD		MILD					SEVERE

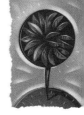

DATE _____

_____

_____
_____
_____
_____
_____
_____
_____

*"When we cling
to pain we end
up punishing
ourselves."*

From **Personhood –
The Art of Being
Fully Human,** by
Leo F. Buscaglia,
PhD, educator
and author

_____
_____
_____
_____
_____
_____
_____
_____
_____
_____
_____
_____
_____

My mood today was:

0	1	2	3	4	5
GOOD					BAD

My level of pain today was:

0	1	2	3	4	5
MILD					SEVERE

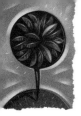

DATE _____

_____
_____
_____
_____
_____
_____
_____

"*Love not what
you are but only
what you may
become.*"

Miguel de Cervantes,
Spanish novelist
and author

_____
_____
_____
_____
_____
_____
_____
_____
_____
_____
_____
_____
_____
_____
_____
_____
_____

			My mood today was:			
0	1	2	3	4	5
GOOD					BAD

			My level of pain today was:			
0	1	2	3	4	5
MILD					SEVERE

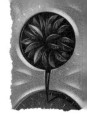

_____

_____

_____

_____

_____

_____

_____

_____

_____

_____

_____

_____

_____

_____

_____

_____

_____

_____

_____

_____

_____

_____

_____

_____

_____

My mood today was:							**My level of pain today was:**					
0	1	2	3	4	5		0	1	2	3	4	5
GOOD					BAD		MILD					SEVERE

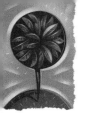

DATE _____

_____

_____
_____
_____
_____
_____
_____
_____
_____
_____
_____
_____
_____
_____
_____
_____
_____
_____
_____
_____
_____
_____
_____
_____
_____

My mood today was:

0	1	2	3	4	5

GOOD ———————————————— BAD

My level of pain today was:

0	1	2	3	4	5

MILD ———————————————— SEVERE

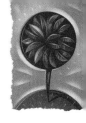

_____

_____

_____

_____

_____

_____

_____

_____

_____

_____

_____

_____

_____

_____

_____

_____

_____

_____

_____

_____

_____

_____

_____

_____

_____

_____

_____

"Every person, all the events of your life are there because you have drawn them there. What you choose to do with them is up to you."

From *Illusions: The Adventures of a Reluctant Messiah,* by Richard Bach

My mood today was:					
0	1	2	3	4	5
GOOD					BAD

My level of pain today was:					
0	1	2	3	4	5
MILD					SEVERE

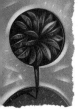

DATE _____

_____
_____
_____
_____
_____
_____
_____
_____
_____
_____
_____
_____
_____
_____
_____
_____
_____
_____
_____
_____
_____
_____
_____
_____
_____

"If I had my life to live over, I would start barefoot earlier in the spring and stay that way later in the fall. I would go to more dances. I would ride more merry-go-rounds. I would pick more daisies."

From the poem
"If I Had My Life to Live Over,"
by Nadine Stair

My mood today was:							My level of pain today was:					
0	1	2	3	4	5		0	1	2	3	4	5
GOOD					BAD		MILD					SEVERE

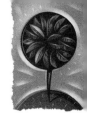

DATE _____

_____

_____
_____
_____
_____
_____
_____
_____
_____
_____
_____
_____
_____
_____
_____
_____
_____
_____
_____
_____
_____
_____
_____
_____
_____
_____
_____
_____

My mood today was:

0	1	2	3	4	5
GOOD					BAD

My level of pain today was:

0	1	2	3	4	5
MILD					SEVERE

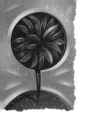

DATE

_____

_____

_____

_____

_____

_____

_____

_____

_____

_____

_____

_____

_____

_____

_____

_____

_____

_____

_____

_____

_____

_____

_____

_____

_____

My mood today was:

0	1	2	3	4	5
GOOD					BAD

My level of pain today was:

0	1	2	3	4	5
MILD					SEVERE

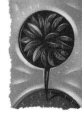

DATE _____

_____

_____
_____
_____
_____
_____
_____

"Never go to a doctor whose office plants have died."

Erma Bombeck,
humor columnist
and author

_____
_____
_____
_____
_____
_____
_____
_____
_____
_____
_____
_____
_____
_____
_____

My mood today was:

0	1	2	3	4	5
GOOD					BAD

My level of pain today was:

0	1	2	3	4	5
MILD					SEVERE

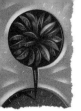

DATE _____

_____

_____

_____

_____

_____

_____

"Your heaviest   _____
artillery will
be your will to   _____
live. Keep that
big gun going."   _____

From *Anatomy* _____
of an Illness:
As Perceived by _____
the Patient, by
Norman Cousins _____

_____

_____

_____

_____

_____

_____

_____

_____

_____

My mood today was:

0	1	2	3	4	5
GOOD					BAD

My level of pain today was:

0	1	2	3	4	5
MILD					SEVERE

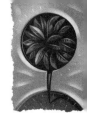

DATE _____

_____

_____
_____
_____
_____
_____
_____
_____
_____
_____
_____
_____
_____
_____
_____
_____
_____
_____
_____
_____
_____
_____
_____
_____
_____
_____
_____
_____

My mood today was:

0	1	2	3	4	5

GOOD ———————————————— BAD

My level of pain today was:

0	1	2	3	4	5

MILD ———————————————— SEVERE

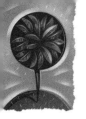

DATE _____

_____
_____
_____
_____
_____
_____
_____
_____
_____
_____
_____
_____
_____
_____
_____
_____
_____
_____
_____
_____
_____
_____
_____
_____

My mood today was:					
0	1	2	3	4	5
GOOD					BAD

My level of pain today was:					
0	1	2	3	4	5
MILD					SEVERE

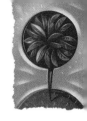

"I'd rather look back on life and say 'I'm sorry I did rather than 'I wish I had.'"

Unknown

My mood today was:

0	1	2	3	4	5

GOOD ———————————————— BAD

My level of pain today was:

0	1	2	3	4	5

MILD ———————————————— SEVERE

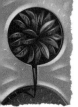

DATE _____

_____

_____

_____

_____

_____

_____

"*Each person
deserves a day
away in which
no problems are
confronted, no
solutions searched
for. Each of us
needs to withdraw
from the cares
which will not
withdraw from us.
A day away acts
as a spring tonic.
It can dispel
rancor, transform
indecision, and
renew the spirit.*"

From *Wouldn't
Take Nothing for
My Journey Now,*
by Maya Angelou,
poet and author

My mood today was:

0	1	2	3	4	5
GOOD					BAD

My level of pain today was:

0	1	2	3	4	5
MILD					SEVERE

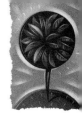

DATE

_____

My mood today was:

0   1   2   3   4   5

GOOD ——————————————— BAD

My level of pain today was:

0   1   2   3   4   5

MILD ——————————————— SEVERE

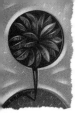

DATE _____

_____

_____

_____

_____

_____

_____

_____

_____

_____

_____

_____

_____

_____

_____

_____

_____

_____

_____

_____

_____

_____

_____

_____

_____

My mood today was:							My level of pain today was:					
0	1	2	3	4	5		0	1	2	3	4	5
GOOD					BAD		MILD					SEVERE

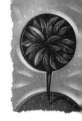

DATE _____

_____

_____

_____

_____

_____

_____

_____

_____

_____   *"It would be nice*
if we could forget
_____   *our troubles as*
easily as we forget
_____   *our blessings."*

_____   Unknown

_____

_____

_____

_____

_____

_____

_____

_____

_____

_____

_____

_____

My mood today was:							**My level of pain today was:**					
0	1	2	3	4	5		0	1	2	3	4	5
GOOD					BAD		MILD					SEVERE

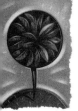

DATE

_____

"Don't just settle
back and say,
'Well, I've got
arthritis and just
can't do anything
about it.' The more
you give in to it,
the worse it gets."

Sarah Cannon
(Minnie Pearl), who
lived with rheuma-
toid arthritis for
25 of her 50 years
in show business,
offering her best
advice. As quoted
in *Arthritis Today,*
March-April 1990

My mood today was:

0	1	2	3	4	5
GOOD					BAD

My level of pain today was:

0	1	2	3	4	5
MILD					SEVERE

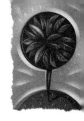

DATE

_____

My mood today was:

0	1	2	3	4	5
GOOD					BAD

My level of pain today was:

0	1	2	3	4	5
MILD					SEVERE

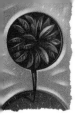

DATE _____

_____
_____
_____
_____
_____
_____
_____
_____
_____
_____
_____
_____
_____
_____
_____
_____
_____
_____
_____
_____
_____
_____
_____
_____

My mood today was:

0	1	2	3	4	5
GOOD					BAD

My level of pain today was:

0	1	2	3	4	5
MILD					SEVERE

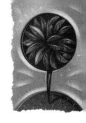

DATE

"*Try to live in the present; don't carry around unnecessary burdens from a yesterday you will not live again or a tomorrow that is not guaranteed.*"

From *The Measure of Our Success*, by Marian Wright Edelman

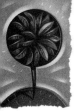

DATE _____

_____

_____

_____

_____

_____

_____

"The goal is a cure.
The goal is to
get up and out of
the wheelchair.
And in the
meantime, you
deal with reality.
But if you don't
have a vision,
nothing happens."

Actor Christopher
Reeve, interviewed
in *Physical Therapy*
magazine, June 1997

My mood today was:					
0	1	2	3	4	5
GOOD					BAD

My level of pain today was:					
0	1	2	3	4	5
MILD					SEVERE

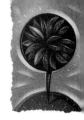

DATE

_____

_____
_____
_____
_____
_____
_____
_____
_____
_____
_____
_____
_____
_____
_____
_____
_____
_____
_____
_____
_____
_____
_____
_____
_____
_____
_____

My mood today was:						My level of pain today was:					
0	1	2	3	4	5	0	1	2	3	4	5
GOOD					BAD	MILD					SEVERE

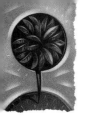

DATE _____

_____
_____
_____
_____
_____
_____
_____
_____
_____
_____
_____
_____
_____
_____
_____
_____
_____
_____
_____
_____
_____
_____
_____
_____
_____
_____
_____

My mood today was:							**My level of pain today was:**					
0	1	2	3	4	5		0	1	2	3	4	5
GOOD					BAD		MILD					SEVERE

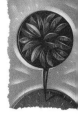

_"If you can talk,
you can sing.
If you can walk,
you can dance."_

African proverb

My mood today was:

0	1	2	3	4	5
GOOD					BAD

My level of pain today was:

0	1	2	3	4	5
MILD					SEVERE

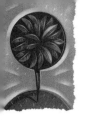

DATE _____

_____

_____

_____

_____

_____

_____

_____

"The journey of 1,000 miles begins with a single step."

Lao Tsu, 6th century
Chinese philosopher

_____

_____

_____

_____

_____

_____

_____

_____

_____

_____

_____

_____

_____

_____

_____

_____

_____

_____

My mood today was:

0	1	2	3	4	5
GOOD					BAD

My level of pain today was:

0	1	2	3	4	5
MILD					SEVERE

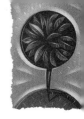

DATE _____

_____

_____
_____
_____
_____
_____
_____
_____
_____
_____
_____
_____
_____
_____
_____
_____
_____
_____
_____
_____
_____
_____
_____
_____
_____
_____
_____

My mood today was:

0	1	2	3	4	5

GOOD ——————————————————— BAD

My level of pain today was:

0	1	2	3	4	5

MILD ——————————————————— SEVERE

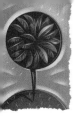

DATE _____

_____

_____

_____

_____

_____

_____

_____

_____

_____

_____

_____

_____

_____

_____

_____

_____

_____

_____

_____

_____

_____

_____

_____

_____

_____

My mood today was:

0	1	2	3	4	5

GOOD ———————————————————— BAD

My level of pain today was:

0	1	2	3	4	5

MILD ———————————————————— SEVERE

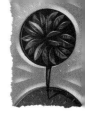

DATE _____

_____

_____
_____
_____
_____
_____
_____
_____
_____
_____
_____
_____
_____
_____
_____
_____
_____
_____
_____
_____
_____
_____
_____
_____
_____
_____

"It feels good to be able to say, 'I've overcome that stage' and to offer your perspective to someone who can't yet see the light at the end of the tunnel. Sometimes you're the one offering encouragement; sometimes you're getting it."

Donna Huser, who has dermatomyositis and rheumatoid arthritis, on arthritis support groups. As quoted in *Arthritis Today*, September-October 1996

My mood today was:

0	1	2	3	4	5
GOOD					BAD

My level of pain today was:

0	1	2	3	4	5
MILD					SEVERE

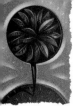

DATE _____

_____

_____

_____

_____

_____

_____

_____

"And as for me,
let what will come,
I can receive no
damage from it,
unless I think it
a calamity; and
it is in my power
to think it none,
if I so decide."

Marcus Aurelius,
Roman emperor
and philosopher

_____

_____

_____

_____

_____

_____

_____

_____

_____

_____

_____

_____

_____

_____

_____

_____

My mood today was:							**My level of pain today was:**					
0	1	2	3	4	5		0	1	2	3	4	5
GOOD					BAD		MILD					SEVERE

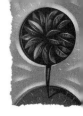

DATE

_____

My mood today was:

| 0 | 1 | 2 | 3 | 4 | 5 |

GOOD ——————————————— BAD

My level of pain today was:

| 0 | 1 | 2 | 3 | 4 | 5 |

MILD ——————————————— SEVERE

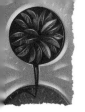

DATE

_____

_____

_____

_____

_____

_____

_____

_____

_____

_____

_____

_____

_____

_____

_____

_____

_____

_____

_____

_____

_____

_____

_____

_____

_____

_____

My mood today was:

0	1	2	3	4	5

GOOD ———————————————— BAD

My level of pain today was:

0	1	2	3	4	5

MILD ———————————————— SEVERE

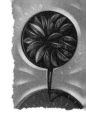

DATE

_____

"*Success is to be
measured not
so much by the
position one has
reached in life,
as by the obstacles
he has overcome
while trying
to succeed.*"

Booker T. Wash-
ington, leader,
inventor, author
and educator

My mood today was:						My level of pain today was:					
0	1	2	3	4	5	0	1	2	3	4	5
GOOD					BAD	MILD					SEVERE

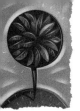

DATE _____

_____

_____

_____

_____

_____

_____

"Stand silently
and watch the
world go by –
and it will."

Unknown

_____

_____

_____

_____

_____

_____

_____

_____

_____

_____

_____

_____

_____

_____

My mood today was:						My level of pain today was:					
0	1	2	3	4	5	0	1	2	3	4	5
GOOD					BAD	MILD					SEVERE

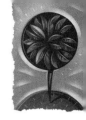

DATE _____

_____

_____
_____
_____
_____
_____
_____
_____
_____
_____
_____
_____
_____
_____
_____
_____
_____
_____
_____
_____
_____
_____
_____
_____
_____
_____
_____

My mood today was:						**My level of pain today was:**					
0	1	2	3	4	5	0	1	2	3	4	5
GOOD					BAD	MILD					SEVERE

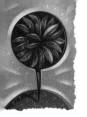

DATE _____

_____
_____
_____
_____
_____
_____
_____
_____
_____
_____
_____
_____
_____
_____
_____
_____
_____
_____
_____
_____
_____
_____
_____
_____
_____

My mood today was:						My level of pain today was:					
0	1	2	3	4	5	0	1	2	3	4	5
GOOD					BAD	MILD					SEVERE

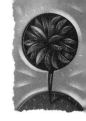

_____

_____

_____

_____

_____

_____

_____

_____   *"Don't compromise*
                                                  yourself. You are
_____   *all you've got."*

_____   Janis Joplin,
                                                  singer/songwriter
_____

_____

_____

_____

_____

_____

_____

_____

_____

_____

_____

_____

_____

My mood today was:

0	1	2	3	4	5
GOOD					BAD

My level of pain today was:

0	1	2	3	4	5
MILD					SEVERE

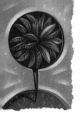

DATE _____

_____
_____
_____
_____
_____
_____

"As human beings
our greatness lies
not so much in be-
ing able to remake
the world – that is
the myth of the
'Atomic Age' – as
in being able to
remake ourselves."

Hindu national
leader Mahatma
Gandhi, quoted in
The Measure of
Our Success, by
Marian Wright
Edelman

_____
_____
_____
_____
_____
_____
_____
_____
_____
_____
_____
_____
_____
_____
_____
_____
_____
_____
_____

My mood today was:							**My level of pain today was:**					
0	1	2	3	4	5		0	1	2	3	4	5
GOOD					BAD		MILD					SEVERE

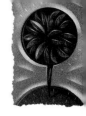

DATE _____

_____

_____

_____

_____

_____

_____

_____

_____

_____

_____

_____

_____

_____

_____

_____

_____

_____

_____

_____

_____

_____

_____

_____

_____

_____

_____

_____

My mood today was:	**My level of pain today was:**
0 1 2 3 4 5	0 1 2 3 4 5
GOOD ———————————— BAD	MILD ———————————— SEVERE

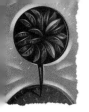

DATE _____

_____

_____

_____

_____

_____

_____

_____

_____

_____

_____

_____

_____

_____

_____

_____

_____

_____

_____

_____

_____

_____

_____

_____

_____

_____

My mood today was:						My level of pain today was:					
0	1	2	3	4	5	0	1	2	3	4	5
GOOD					BAD	MILD					SEVERE

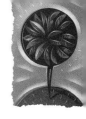

"For the day will come when we are able to contain the wolf [of arthritis] and it will no longer wreak havoc with the lives of our children. ...It is our mission to keep the home fires burning, to keep a light in the window, to keep supper warm, and, without fail, to provide hope, love and support. ...For after all they are our children."

Janet Austin, PhD, vice president of the Arthritis Foundation's American Juvenile Arthritis Organization (AJAO) and Arthritis-Related Groups. Austin has had rheumatoid arthritis since age 16.

My mood today was:

0	1	2	3	4	5

GOOD ——————————————— BAD

My level of pain today was:

0	1	2	3	4	5

MILD ——————————————— SEVERE

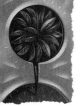

DATE _____

_____
_____
_____
_____
_____
_____
_____

"…sometimes the best outcome is being able to see that there are things in life which are neither understandable or acceptable – and in understanding, and accepting that, real peace can come."

From *Life Is Goodbye, Life Is Hello: Grieving Well Through All Kinds of Loss,* by Alla Renee Bozarth, PhD

_____
_____
_____
_____
_____
_____
_____
_____
_____
_____
_____
_____
_____
_____
_____

My mood today was:

0	1	2	3	4	5
GOOD					BAD

My level of pain today was:

0	1	2	3	4	5
MILD					SEVERE

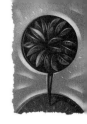

_____
DATE

_____

_____

_____

_____

_____

_____

_____

_____

_____

_____

_____

_____

_____

_____

_____

_____

_____

_____

_____

_____

_____

_____

_____

_____

_____

_____

	My mood today was:			**My level of pain today was:**	
0 1 2 3 4 5			0 1 2 3 4 5		
GOOD — BAD			MILD — SEVERE		

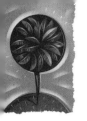

DATE _____

_____

_____

_____

_____

_____

_____

_____

_____

_____

_____

_____

_____

_____

_____

_____

_____

_____

_____

_____

_____

_____

_____

_____

_____

My mood today was:	My level of pain today was:
0 1 2 3 4 5	0 1 2 3 4 5
GOOD ———————— BAD	MILD ———————— SEVERE

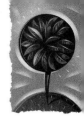

DATE _____

_____

_____

_____

_____

_____

_____

_____

_____   *"We tend not to choose the un-known...and yet it is the un-known with all its disappoint-ments and sur-prises that is most enriching."*

_____

_____   From **Gift from the Sea,** by Anne Morrow Lindbergh

_____

_____

_____

_____

_____

_____

_____

_____

_____

_____

_____

My mood today was:

0	1	2	3	4	5
GOOD					BAD

My level of pain today was:

0	1	2	3	4	5
MILD					SEVERE

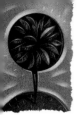

DATE _____

_____
_____
_____
_____
_____
_____
_____

"Keep your face
to the sunshine
and you cannot
see the shadows."

_____
_____
_____

A favorite quote of
teenager Stephanie
Nelson of Sterling,
Colo., who has fibro-
myalgia and rheuma-
toid arthritis. From
Your Personal Guide
to Living Well with
Fibromyalgia.

_____
_____
_____
_____
_____
_____
_____
_____
_____
_____
_____
_____
_____
_____

My mood today was:						**My level of pain today was:**					
0	1	2	3	4	5	0	1	2	3	4	5
GOOD					BAD	MILD					SEVERE

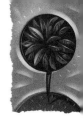

DATE _____

_____

_____

_____

_____

_____

_____

_____

_____

_____

_____

_____

_____

_____

_____

_____

_____

_____

_____

_____

_____

_____

_____

_____

_____

_____

_____

My mood today was:

0	1	2	3	4	5
GOOD					BAD

My level of pain today was:

0	1	2	3	4	5
MILD					SEVERE

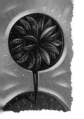

DATE _____

_____

_____

_____

_____

_____

_____

_____

_____

_____

_____

_____

_____

_____

_____

_____

_____

_____

_____

_____

_____

_____

_____

_____

_____

_____

My mood today was:	My level of pain today was:
0　1　2　3　4　5	0　1　2　3　4　5
GOOD ———————— BAD	MILD ———————— SEVERE

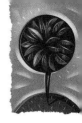

DATE _____

_____

_____

_____

_____

_____

_____

_____   *"If you have built*
                                                  castles in the air,
_____   *your work need*
                                                  not be lost; that
_____   *is where they*
                                                  should be. Now
_____   *put foundations*
                                                  under them."
_____
                                                  Henry David
_____   Thoreau, naturalist
                                                  and writer
_____

_____

_____

_____

_____

_____

_____

_____

_____

My mood today was:							My level of pain today was:					
0	1	2	3	4	5		0	1	2	3	4	5
GOOD					BAD		MILD					SEVERE

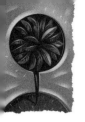

DATE _____

_____
_____
_____
_____
_____
_____
_____
_____

"Don't worry.
Be happy."

Bobby McFerrin,
singer/songwriter

_____
_____
_____
_____
_____
_____
_____
_____
_____
_____
_____
_____
_____
_____

My mood today was:

0	1	2	3	4	5
GOOD					BAD

My level of pain today was:

0	1	2	3	4	5
MILD					SEVERE

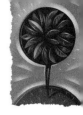

DATE

_____

My mood today was:

0	1	2	3	4	5
GOOD					BAD

My level of pain today was:

0	1	2	3	4	5
MILD					SEVERE

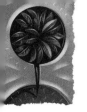

DATE

_____

_____

_____

_____

_____

_____

_____

_____

_____

_____

_____

_____

_____

_____

_____

_____

_____

_____

_____

_____

_____

_____

_____

_____

My mood today was:

0	1	2	3	4	5
GOOD					BAD

My level of pain today was:

0	1	2	3	4	5
MILD					SEVERE

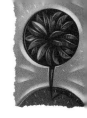

"*These the old blues
and I sing 'em,
sing 'em, sing 'em.
Just like any
woman do.
My life ain't
done yet
Naw…My song
ain't through.*"

From the poem "Any
Woman's Blues", by
writer Sherley Anne
Williams, as appeared
in *Render Me My
Song* by Sandi Russell

My mood today was:

| 0 | 1 | 2 | 3 | 4 | 5 |

GOOD — BAD

My level of pain today was:

| 0 | 1 | 2 | 3 | 4 | 5 |

MILD — SEVERE

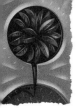

DATE

"*Every life is a play in which the lead character is center stage – and the lead character in your life is you.*"

Sonya Friedman,
1986 Academy
Award-nominated
documentarian

My mood today was:

0	1	2	3	4	5
GOOD					BAD

My level of pain today was:

0	1	2	3	4	5
MILD					SEVERE

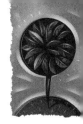

DATE _____

_____

_____

_____

_____

_____

_____

_____

_____

_____

_____

_____

_____

_____

_____

_____

_____

_____

_____

_____

_____

_____

_____

_____

_____

_____

_____

_____

_____

	My mood today was:							**My level of pain today was:**				
0	1	2	3	4	5		0	1	2	3	4	5
GOOD					BAD		MILD					SEVERE

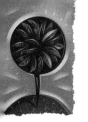

DATE

_____

My mood today was:

0	1	2	3	4	5
GOOD					BAD

My level of pain today was:

0	1	2	3	4	5
MILD					SEVERE

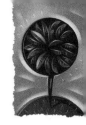

DATE

"Be bold. If you're going to make an error, make a doozy, and don't be afraid to hit the ball."

Billie Jean King, professional tennis champion

My mood today was:

0	1	2	3	4	5
GOOD					BAD

My level of pain today was:

0	1	2	3	4	5
MILD					SEVERE

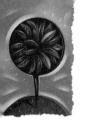

DATE _____

_____
_____
_____
_____
_____
_____
_____

"Success is more attitude than aptitude."

Unknown

_____
_____
_____
_____
_____
_____
_____
_____
_____
_____
_____
_____
_____
_____
_____
_____
_____
_____

My mood today was:

0	1	2	3	4	5
GOOD					BAD

My level of pain today was:

0	1	2	3	4	5
MILD					SEVERE

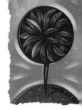

DATE _____

_____

_____

_____

_____

_____

_____

_____

_____

_____

_____

_____

_____

_____

_____

_____

_____

_____

_____

_____

_____

_____

_____

_____

_____

_____

_____

My mood today was:

0	1	2	3	4	5

GOOD ——————————————— BAD

My level of pain today was:

0	1	2	3	4	5

MILD ——————————————— SEVERE

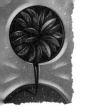

DATE _____

_____

_____

_____

_____

_____

_____

_____

_____

_____

_____

_____

_____

_____

_____

_____

_____

_____

_____

_____

_____

_____

_____

_____

My mood today was:

0   1   2   3   4   5

GOOD ——————————————— BAD

My level of pain today was:

0   1   2   3   4   5

MILD ——————————————— SEVERE

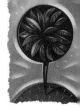

DATE

_____

"Some see things
as they are and
ask why. I dream
things that
never were and
ask why not."

Robert F. Kennedy,
United States Senator

My mood today was:

0	1	2	3	4	5
GOOD					BAD

My level of pain today was:

0	1	2	3	4	5
MILD					SEVERE

RESOURCES

The Arthritis Foundation is the source of help and hope for nearly 40 million Americans who have arthritis, rheumatic diseases and related musculoskeletal conditions. Founded in 1948, the Arthritis Foundation is the only national, voluntary health organization that works for all people affected by any of the more than 100 forms of arthritis or related conditions. Volunteers in chapters nationwide help to support research, professional and community education programs, services for people with arthritis, government advocacy and fund-raising activities.

The American Juvenile Arthritis Organization (AJAO) comprises children, parents, teachers and others concerned specifically about juvenile arthritis. A council of the Arthritis Foundation, AJAO focuses its efforts on the problems related to arthritis in children.

The mission of the Arthritis Foundation is twofold: to support research to find the cure for and prevention of arthritis, and to improve the quality of life for those affected by arthritis. Public contributions enable the Arthritis Foundation to fulfill this mission – in fact, at least 80 cents of every dollar donated to the Arthritis Foundation directly funds research and program services.

How the Arthritis Foundation Helps

Arthritis doesn't have to rob you of the activities you enjoy most. While research holds the key to future cures or preventions for arthritis, equally important is improving the quality of life for people with arthritis today. Your local Arthritis Foundation office has information, classes and other services to help you take charge of your arthritis. The Arthritis Foundation has more than 150 local offices across the United States. To find the office near you, and to determine which of the following resources are available through your nearest chapter, call 800/283-7800.

Medical and Self-Care Programs

Physician referral – Most Arthritis Foundation chapters can give you a list of doctors in your area who specialize in the evaluation and treatment of arthritis and arthritis-related conditions.

Exercise programs – Recreational in nature, these are developed, coordinated and sponsored by the Arthritis Foundation. All have specially trained instructors. They include:

- Joint Efforts – This arthritis movement program teaches gentle, undemanding movement exercises for people with arthritis, including those who use walkers and wheelchairs. Joint Efforts is designed to encourage movement and socialization among older adults and to help decrease pain, stiffness and depression.

- PACE® (People with Arthritis Can Exercise) – PACE® is an exercise program that uses gentle activities to help increase joint flexibility, range of motion and stamina, and to help maintain muscle strength. Two videotapes showing basic and advanced levels of the program are available from your local chapter for preview or for practice at home. To purchase the videos, call 800/207-8633.

- Arthritis Foundation Aquatic Program – Originally co-developed by the YMCA and the Arthritis Foundation, this water exercise program helps relieve the strain on muscles and joints for people with arthritis. The PEP (Pool Exercise Program) videotape shows how to exercise on your own. To order the video, call 800/207-8633.

Educational and Support Groups

Arthritis Foundation Support Groups – These are mutual-support groups that provide opportunities for discussion and problem solving. They are usually formed by people with arthritis and/or their family members who wish to meet with their peers for mutual assistance in satisfying common needs and in overcoming problems related to arthritis.

Classes/courses – Formal group meetings help people with various forms of arthritis gain the knowledge, skills and confidence they need to actively manage their conditions. Courses focus on proper exercises, medications, relaxation techniques, pain management, dealing with depression, nutrition, nontraditional treatments and doctor-patient relations. The classes include:

- Arthritis Self-Help Course
- Fibromyalgia Self-Help Course
- Systemic Lupus Erythematosus Self-Help Course.

Reliable Information at Your Fingertips

Information hotline – The Arthritis Foundation is the expert on arthritis and is only a phone call away. Call 800/283-7800 toll-free for automated information on arthritis 24 hours a day. Trained volunteers and staff are also available at your local Arthritis Foundation to answer your questions or to send you a list of physicians in your area who specialize in arthritis.

Arthritis Foundation Web site – Information about arthritis is available 24 hours a day to Internet users via the Arthritis Foundation's site on the World Wide Web. The address for the Web site is http://www.arthritis.org.

Publications – A number of publications are available to educate people with arthritis, their families and friends about important considerations such as medications, exercise, diet, pain management and stress management, to name a few.

- Books – Self-help books by the Arthritis Foundation – including *Your Personal Guide to Living Well with Fibromyalgia, 250 Tips for Making Life with Arthritis Easier* and *Arthritis 101: Questions You Have. Answers You Need.* – are available to help you learn more about your condition and how to manage it. Check your local bookstores, call your local Arthritis Foundation chapter, or order a book through the Arthritis Foundation by calling 800/207-8633.

- Booklets – More than 60 booklets and brochures provide information on the many arthritis-related diseases and conditions, medications, how to work with your doctor, and how to care for yourself. Single copies are available free of charge. Call 800/283-7800 for a free listing of booklets on arthritis.

- *Arthritis Today* – The award-winning bimonthly magazine *Arthritis Today* gives you the latest information on research, new treatments and tips from experts and readers to help you manage arthritis. Each issue also brings you a variety of helpful and interesting articles covering diet and nutrition, exercise tips and ways you can make your life with arthritis easier and more rewarding. You'll also have access to a wide range of local chapter activities. A one-year subscription to *Arthritis Today* is yours free when you become a member of the Arthritis Foundation. Annual membership helps fund research to find cures for arthritis. Call 800/933-0032 for membership and subscription information. *Arthritis Today* is also available on selected newsstands.

Audiovisual libraries – Available either on loan or for purchase, a number of audiocassettes and videos cover a variety of topics from exercise to relaxation. Call your local chapter for a listing of titles, prices and availabilities.

Public forums – Educational programs are presented to the community on various requested topics.

Professional publications – A number of education materials on arthritis geared to the health-care professional are available through the Arthritis Foundation. These materials, including the *Bulletin on the Rheumatic Diseases,* a newsletter published eight times a year, and the 513-page *Primer on the Rheumatic Diseases* (also on CD-ROM) which is published every five years, are available by calling 800/207-8633.

Remember the Arthritis Foundation in Your Will

The mission of the Arthritis Foundation is to support arthritis research and to improve the quality of life for those affected by it. Planned giving is an important part of this mission. The Foundation's planned giving department offers a wide variety of gift planning options, including estate gifts and gifts that provide donors with lifetime income. We hope that you decide to include a gift to the Foundation in your will. For more information, call the Arthritis Foundation's planned giving department at 404/872-7100.

Arthritis Foundation
1330 West Peachtree St.
Atlanta, GA 30309
404/872-7100
http://www.arthritis.org

ADDITIONAL RESOURCES

ADDITIONAL RESOURCES

ADDITIONAL RESOURCES

ACKNOWLEDGMENTS

The quotes in this journal were compiled from a variety of sources. Following is a list of these sources, in the order that they appear in the journal.

Reprinted from *Living Faith,* by Jimmy Carter, New York, NY, Random House, Inc. 1996.

Reprinted from *Gather Together In My Name,* by Maya Angelou, New York, NY, Random House, Inc. 1974.

Reprinted with permission from *To Lead Is To Serve,* by Shar McBee. Copyright 1994 by Shar McBee.

Reprinted from *The Diary of a Young Girl: The Definitive Edition,* by Anne Frank. Otto H. Frank and Mirjam Pressler, Editors, translated by Susan Massotty. Translation copyright 1995 by Doubleday, a division of Bantam Doubleday Dell Publishing Group, Inc. Used by permission of Doubleday, a division of Bantam Doubleday Dell Publishing Group, Inc.

Reprinted from *Where the Wild Things Are,* by Maurice Sendak. Copyright 1963 by Maurice Sendak. Used by permission of HarperCollins Publishers.

Reprinted from *Life's Answers,* by Charles M. Schulz. Copyright 1996 United Features Syndicate.

Reprinted from *Successful Living With Chronic Illness,* copyright 1994 by The Lupus Foundation of America, Inc., Greater Atlanta Chapter. Avery Publishing Group, Garden City Park, New York. Reprinted by permission.

Reprinted from *Inspiration for Living* by Beth Mende Conny. Used by permission of Peter Pauper Press Inc., White Plains, NY. 1992

Reprinted from *Markings,* by Dag Hammarskjold, New York, NY, Random House, Inc. 1966.

Reprinted from *Bird by Bird,* by Anne Lamott, New York, NY, Pantheon Books. 1994.

Reprinted from *Composing A Life,* by Mary Catherine Bateson. Copyright 1989 by Mary Catherine Bateson. Used by permission of Grove/Atlantic, Inc.

Reprinted from *Oh, The Places You'll Go,* by Dr. Seuss. TM and copyright 1990 by Dr. Seuss Enterprises, L.P. Reprinted by permission of Random House, Inc.

Reprinted from *Personhood – The Art of Being Fully Human,* by Dr. Leo Buscaglia, Ph.D., Copyright 1978, by Leo F. Buscaglia, Inc. Published by Slack, Inc.

Reprinted from *Illusions: The Adventures of a Reluctant Messiah,* by Richard Bach. Copyright 1997 by Richard Bach and Leslie Parrish-Bach. Used by permission of Delacorte Press, a division of Bantam Doubleday Dell Publishing Group, Inc.

Excerpts from "Oppressed Hair Puts A Ceiling On The Brain" and "Journal (June, September 1987)" in *Living By the Word: Selected Writings 1973-1987,* copyright by Alice Walker, reprinted by permission of Harcourt Brace & Company.

Reprinted from *Anatomy of an Illness: As Perceived by the Patient,* by Norman Cousins, New York, NY, W. W. Norton & Company. 1979.

Reprinted from *Wouldn't Take Nothing for My Journey Now,* by Maya Angelou, New York, NY, Random House, Inc. 1993.

Christopher Reeve. Reprinted from *Physical Therapy* magazine, Alexandria, VA, American Physical Therapy Association. June 1997.

Reprinted from *The Measure of Our Success,* by Marian Wright Edelman, Beacon Press. 1992.

Reprinted from *Life is Goodbye/Life is Hello: Grieving Well Through All Kinds of Loss,* by Alla Renee Bozarth, Ph.D., revised edition, Hazelden Educational Services. 1986.

Reprinted from *Gift From the Sea,* by Anne Morrow Lindbergh, New York, NY, Pantheon Books. 1995.

Sherley Anne Williams, "Any Woman's Blues" from *The Peacock Poems,* copyright 1975 by Sherley Williams, Wesleyan University Press. Used by permission of University Press of New England.

Reprinted from *Secrets of Emotional Healing,* by J. Donald Walters, Crystal Clarity, Publishers. 1993.